EAT RIGHT FOR BLOOD TYPE AB

INDIVIDUAL FOOD, DRINK AND SUPPLEMENT LISTS

from

EAT RIGHT
FR
YOUR TYPE

Dr. Peter J. D'Adamo
with Catherine Whitney

PENGUIN BOOKS

PENGUIN BOOKS

Published by the Penguin Group
Penguin Books Ltd, 80 Strand, London WC2R 0RL, England
Penguin Group (USA) Inc., 375 Hudson Street, New York, New York 10014, USA
Penguin Group (Canada), 90 Eglinton Avenue East, Suite 700, Toronto, Ontario,
Canada M4P 2Y3 (a division of Pearson Penguin Canada Inc.)
Penguin Ireland, 25 St Stephen's Green, Dublin 2, Ireland (a division of Penguin Books Ltd)
Penguin Group (Australia), 250 Camberwell Road,
Camberwell, Victoria 3124, Australia (a division of Pearson Australia Group Pty Ltd)
Penguin Books India Pvt Ltd, 11 Community Centre, Panchsheel Park, New Delhi – 110 017, India
Penguin Group (NZ), 67 Apollo Drive, Rosedale, North Shore 0632, New Zealand
(a division of Pearson New Zealand Ltd)
Penguin Books (South Africa) (Pty) Ltd, 24 Sturdee Avenue, Rosebank, Johannesburg 2196, South Africa

Penguin Books Ltd, Registered Offices: 80 Strand, London WC2R 0RL, England

www.penguin.com

First published in the United States of America by The Berkley Publishing Group 2002
First published in Great Britain in Penguin Books 2003
Reissued in this edition 2011

010

ISBN: 978-0-241-95439-3

www.greenpenguin.co.uk

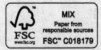

*To Blood Type ABs of the
Twenty-first Century, that you may fully realize
your remarkable heritage.*

Contents

Acknowledgments

There are many people to thank, as no scientific pursuit is solitary. Along the way, I have been driven, inspired, and supported by all of the people who placed their confidence in me. In particular, I give deep thanks to my wife, Martha, for her love and friendship; my daughters, Claudia and Emily, for the joy they bring me; and my parents, James D'Adamo, Sr., N.D., and Christl, for teaching me to trust in my intuition.

I am also more grateful than I can express to:

Catherine Whitney, my writer, and her partner, Paul Krafin, who have transformed complex scientific ideas into accessible principles of everyday life;

My literary agent, Janis Vallely, whose commitment and wisdom are a continuing aid and inspiration;

Amy Hertz, my editor at Riverhead/Putnam, whose

vision and care have turned the blood type science into a meaningful mainstream program;

Jane Dystel, Catherine's literary agent, whose advice has been welcome;

Heidi Merritt, whose devotion and attention to detail have brought the manuscript closer to perfection;

My staff at 2009 Summer Street for their dedication and support, and the hardworking staff at 5 Brook Street;

All of the wonderful patients who in their quest for health and happiness chose to honor me with their trust.

What Type ABs Are Saying About the Diet

Eileen M., 31

"The biggest change for me since going on the Type AB Diet has been the complete balancing of my blood sugar. Before the diet, I had trouble eating any fruit because it would just send my blood sugar on a roller-coaster ride. Now, as long as I follow the diet, my blood sugar is beautifully balanced and I have twice the energy. Another side benefit is that the appearance of my hands and nails has dramatically improved."

James M., 40

"When I went on the Type AB Diet and completely eliminated red meat, my energy levels increased dramatically. Along with renewed energy, I found that I was in a better mood and my mind was sharper. I wasn't really overweight, but the eight-pound weight loss has been a nice side effect. I haven't felt so good in years."

Mary K., 35

"I have suffered from fibromyalgia for several years. After six months on the Type AB Diet, all of my symptoms have been reduced. I have much less pain, more energy, and my resistance to viruses seems better. I've also lost 25 pounds. Before I started this diet I was beginning to think I would never feel right again. I have a whole new lease on life."

Sandra S., 55

"I had been taking a thyroid hormone for about 10 years, but after eight months on the Type AB Diet I was able to discontinue it. I'm doing great. I have also noticed a big improvement in my energy levels. I no longer feel as though I carry a two-ton weight around all the time. I feel like a normal person—something I haven't experienced in many years."

Martha B., 45

"I have been struggling with high cholesterol for several years. No diet that I tried reduced it. In fact, the diet my doctor put me on actually raised my cholesterol. After only a few months on the Type AB Diet, my LDL cholesterol went from 210 to 140, and my total cholesterol is at 170. I almost can't believe it, and my doctor is amazed, too. I'll be on this diet for life."

Ted M., 33

"On the Type AB Diet I have dropped body fat considerably. I went from a 36-inch waist to 30–32-inch waist. I can see my abs again!"

A Message for Type ABs

Dear Type AB Reader,

This special format book, Eat Right 4 Type AB, *focuses on the principles and strategies of the Blood Type Diet as they apply to you. If you are new to the diet, you'll find this book to be a simple, accessible beginner's guide that will get you started on the basics. If you are already following the diet and have read the comprehensive series (*Eat Right 4 Your Type, Cook Right 4 Your Type, *and* Live Right 4 Your Type*), you'll find this book useful as a quick and portable reference guide for your diet.*

Since the introduction of the Blood Type Diet five years ago, I have received tens of thousands of testimonials from people all over the world. Many of them are from Type ABs who have overcome chronic health problems, serious illnesses, or lifelong struggles with weight

merely by eating and living in accordance with the ge-
netic signals of their blood type. A growing body of re-
search supports the conclusion that our individual
differences do matter when it comes to making strategic
health and lifestyle decisions.

I sincerely hope that you will join other Type ABs who
have had success with this plan. I invite you to share in
experiencing the renewed sense of well-being and good
health that have become reliable hallmarks of the Type
AB Diet.

Peter J. D'Adamo, N.D.

IMPORTANT NOTE

The contents of this book have been abridged to provide only the most basic information concerning the Blood Type Diet. To gain the full therapeutic benefit of the diet, it is important that you read Dr. D'Adamo's complete research and prescriptive advice as it appears in his three books, *Eat Right 4 Your Type, Cook Right 4 Your Type,* and *Live Right 4 Your Type*. These books include extensive details that will help you fully understand the important role your blood type plays in determining diet, exercise, health, disease, longevity, physical vitality, and emotional stability.

The Blood Type–Diet Connection

The connection between blood type and diet is a new idea for most people, but they often find that it answers some of their most perplexing questions. We have long realized that there was a missing link in our comprehension of the process that leads either to the path of wellness or the path of disease. There had to be a reason why there were so many paradoxes in dietary studies and disease survival. Blood type analysis has given us a way to explain those paradoxes.

Blood types are as fundamental as creation itself. In the masterful logic of nature, the four blood types follow an unbroken trail from the earliest moment of human creation to the present day. They are the signatures of our ancient ancestors on the indestructible parchment of history. As Blood Type AB, you carry the genetic blend of your Type AB ancestors, incorporating the characteristics of both Type A and Type B. The Type AB gene, still only 1,000 years old, enabled your ancestors to make the transition to modern times.

Your blood type is the key to your body's entire immune system, and as such is the essential defining factor in your health profile. Your blood type antigen serves as the guardian at the gate, creating antibodies to ward off dangerous interlopers. When an antibody encounters the antigen of a microbial invader, a reaction called "agglutination" (literally, gluing) occurs. The antibody attaches to the viral antigen and makes it very sticky. When cells, viruses, parasites, and bacteria are agglutinated, they stick together and clump up, which makes the job of their disposal all the easier.

But there is much more to the agglutination story. Scientists have learned that many foods agglutinate the cells of certain blood types but not others, meaning that a food that may be harmful to the cells of one blood type may be beneficial to the cells of another.

A chemical reaction occurs between your blood and the foods that you eat. This reaction is part of your genetic inheritance. We know this because of a factor called "lectins." Lectins, abundant and diverse proteins found in foods, have agglutinating properties that affect your blood. Lectins are a powerful way for organisms in nature to attach themselves to other organisms in nature. Often, the lectins used by viruses or bacteria can be blood type specific, making them a stickier pest for a person of that blood type. Furthermore, when you eat a food containing protein lectins that are incompatible with your blood type antigen, the lectins target an organ or bodily system (kidneys, liver, brain, stomach, etc.) and begin to agglutinate blood cells in that area. For example, a lectin in lima beans cross-reacts with Type AB blood, targeting digestive enzymes and interfering with insulin production.

The Type AB Diet is a way to restore the natural protective functions of your immune system, reset your metabolic clock, and clear your blood of dangerous agglutinating lectins. Depending on the severity of the condition, and the level of compliance with the plan, every person will realize some benefits from this diet.

THE TYPE AB DIET BASICS

Blood Type AB is less than a thousand years old, rare (2 to 5 percent of the population), and biologically complex. Since you carry both the A and the B antigens, your optimal dietary strategy incorporates both the vegetarian sensibilities of Type A and the meat and dairy needs of Type B. In proper balance, this dietary mix helps keep Type ABs lean, strong, and healthy. The Type AB Diet works because you are able to follow a clear, logical, scientifically researched and certified dietary blueprint based on your cellular profile.

Your diet is organized into fourteen food groups:

Meats and Poultry	Vegetables
Seafood	Fruits
Eggs and Dairy	Juices and Fluids
Oils and Fats	Spices
Nuts and Seeds	Condiments
Beans and Legumes	Herbs and Herbal Teas
Grains, Breads and Pasta	Miscellaneous Beverages

Within each group, food is divided into three categories: HIGHLY BENEFICIAL, NEUTRAL and AVOID. Think of the categories this way:

- **HIGHLY BENEFICIAL** is a food that acts like a **MEDICINE**.

- **AVOID** is a food that acts like a **POISON**.

- **NEUTRAL** is a food that acts like a **FOOD**.

The Type AB Diet includes a wide variety of foods, so don't worry about limitations. When possible, show preference for the Highly Beneficial foods over the Neutral foods, but feel free to enjoy the Neutral foods that suit you; they won't harm you and they contain nutrients that are necessary for a balanced diet.

At the top of each food category, you will see a chart that looks something like this (note that the frequency is sometimes weekly, sometimes daily):

BLOOD TYPE AB		Weekly, if your ancestry is . . .		
	PORTION	AFRICAN	CAUCASIAN	ASIAN
All seafood	4–6 oz.	1–4 x	3–5 x	4–6 x

The portion suggestions according to ancestry are not meant as firm rules. My purpose here is to present a way to fine-tune your diet even more, using what is known about the particulars of your ancestry. Although peoples of different races and cultures may share a blood type, they don't always have the same frequency of the gene. There are also geographic and cultural variations, as well as typical differences in the size and weight of various peoples. Use the refinements if you think they're helpful; ignore them if you find that they're not. In any case, try to formulate your own plan for portion sizes.

CHAPTER ONE

Meats and Poultry

BLOOD TYPE AB		Weekly, if your ancestry is . . .		
	PORTION	AFRICAN	CAUCASIAN	ASIAN
Lean red meats	4–6 oz.	2–3 x	1–3 x	1–3 x
Poultry	(men)			
	2–5 oz.	0–2 x	0–2 x	0–2 x
	(women and children)			

Type ABs need to limit the amount of meat you eat, since you do not produce enough stomach acid to effectively digest too much animal protein. The key for you is portion size and frequency. Give preference to lamb, mutton, rabbit, and turkey over beef. Avoid chicken. It contains a lectin that interferes with Type AB digestion.

HIGHLY BENEFICIAL

Lamb	Rabbit
Mutton	Turkey

NEUTRAL

Liver	Pheasant
Ostrich	

AVOID

Bacon	Heart/Sweetbreads
Beef	Horse
Buffalo	Partridge
Chicken	Pork
Cornish hen	Quail
Duck	Squab
Goose	Squirrel
Grouse	Turtle
Guinea hen	Veal
Ham	Venison

CHAPTER TWO

Seafood

BLOOD TYPE AB		Weekly, if your ancestry is . . .		
	PORTION	AFRICAN	CAUCASIAN	ASIAN
All seafood	4–6 oz.	3–5 x	3–5 x	4–6 x

There is a wide variety of excellent seafood for Type ABs, and it should be a staple of your diet. If you have a family history of breast cancer, introduce snails into your menus. The edible snail, *Helix pomatia,* contains a powerful lectin that specifically agglutinates mutated A-like cells for two of the most common forms of breast cancer. This is a positive kind of agglutination; the snail lectin gets rid of sick cells.

HIGHLY BENEFICIAL

Cod	Mackerel
Grouper	Mahimahi

HIGHLY BENEFICIAL (CONTINUED)

Monkfish	Salmon
Pickerel	Sardine
Pike	Shad
Porgy	Snail (*helix pomatia/ escargot*)
Red snapper	Sturgeon
Sailfish	Tuna

NEUTRAL

Abalone	Cusk
Bluefish	Drum
Bullhead	Halfmoon fish
Butterfish	Harvest fish
Carp	Herring (fresh)
Catfish	Mullet
Caviar	Muskelunge
Chub	Mussels
Croaker	Opaleye fish

NEUTRAL (CONTINUED)

Orange roughy	Smelt
Parrot fish	Snapper
Perch (all types)	Squid (calamari)
Pollack	Sucker
Pompano	Sunfish
Rosefish	Swordfish
Scallop	Tilapia
Scrod	Tilefish
Scup	Weakfish
Shark	Whitefish

AVOID

Anchovy	Conch
Barracuda	Crab
Bass (all types)	Crayfish
Beluga	Eel
Clam	Flounder

AVOID (CONTINUED)

Frog	Oysters
Haddock	Salmon roe
Hake	Shrimp
Halibut	Sole (all types)
Herring (pickled)	Trout (all types)
Lobster	Whiting
Lox	Yellowtail
Octopus	

CHAPTER THREE

Eggs and Dairy

BLOOD TYPE AB		Weekly, if your ancestry is . . .		
	PORTION	AFRICAN	CAUCASIAN	ASIAN
Eggs	1 egg	2–6 x	3–4 x	2–3 x
Cheese	2 oz.	2–3 x	3–4 x	3–4 x
Yogurt	4–6 oz.	1–4 x	2–3 x	1–4 x
Milk	4–6 oz.	1–2 x	1–3 x	0–2 x

Type ABs benefit from dairy foods, especially cultured and soured products—buttermilk, yogurt, kefir, and sour cream—which are easily digested. The primary factor you have to watch out for is excessive mucus production. If you have respiratory problems, sinus attacks, or ear infections, cut back on dairy foods. Eggs are a very good source of protein for Type ABs.

HIGHLY BENEFICIAL

Cottage cheese	Kefir
Egg white (chicken)	Mozzarella
Farmer cheese	Ricotta
Feta	Sour cream (low fat)
Goat cheese	Yogurt
Goat milk	

NEUTRAL

Casein	Goose egg
Cheddar	Gouda
Colby	Gruyère
Cream cheese	Jarlsberg
Edam	Milk (cow, skim, 1percent, 2 percent)
Egg yolk (chicken)	Monterey jack
Emmenthal	Muenster
Ghee (clarified butter)	Neufchâtel

NEUTRAL (CONTINUED)

Paneer	String cheese
Quail egg	Swiss
Quark cheese	Whey

AVOID

American cheese	Half & Half
Blue cheese	Ice cream
Brie	Milk (cow, whole)
Butter	Parmesan
Buttermilk	Provolone
Camembert	Sherbet
Duck egg	

CHAPTER FOUR

Oils and Fats

BLOOD TYPE AB		Weekly, if your ancestry is . . .		
	PORTION	AFRICAN	CAUCASIAN	ASIAN
Oils	1 tablespoon	4–7 x	5–8 x	5–7 x

Type ABs should use olive oil rather than animal fats, hydrogenated vegetable fats, or other vegetable oils. Olive oil is a monounsaturated fat, which is believed to contribute to lower blood cholesterol.

HIGHLY BENEFICIAL

Olive	Walnut

NEUTRAL

Almond	Borage
Black currant seed	Canola

NEUTRAL (CONTINUED)

Castor	Peanut
Cod liver	Soy
Evening primrose	Wheat germ
Linseed (flaxseed)	

AVOID

Coconut	Safflower
Corn	Sesame
Cottonseed	Sunflower

CHAPTER FIVE

Nuts and Seeds

BLOOD TYPE AB		Weekly, if your ancestry is . . .		
	PORTION	AFRICAN	CAUCASIAN	ASIAN
Nuts and seeds	Small handful	2–4 x	2–4 x	2–3 x
Nut butters	1–2 tablespoons	3–6 x	3–6 x	3–6 x

Nuts and seeds present a mixed picture for Type ABs. Eat them in small amounts and with caution. Although they can be a good supplementary protein source, all seeds contain the insulin-inhibiting lectins that make them a problem for Type ABs. On the other hand, peanuts are powerful immune boosters for you.

HIGHLY BENEFICIAL

Chestnut	Peanut butter
Peanut	Walnut

NEUTRAL

Almond	Hickory
Almond butter	Lychee
Almond cheese	Macadamia
Almond milk	Pecan/pecan butter
Beechnut	Pignola (pine nut)
Brazil nut	Pistachio
Cashew/cashew butter	Safflower seed
Flaxseed (linseed)	

AVOID

Filbert (hazelnut)	Sesame seed
Poppy seed	Sesame butter (tahini)
Pumpkin seed	Sunflower seed/butter

CHAPTER SIX

Beans and Legumes

BLOOD TYPE AB		Weekly, if your ancestry is . . .		
	PORTION	AFRICAN	CAUCASIAN	ASIAN
Beans and legumes	1 cup, dry	3–5 x	2–3 x	4–6 x

Beans and legumes are another mixed bag for Type ABs. Lentils are known to contain cancer-fighting antioxidants. On the other hand, kidney and lima beans slow insulin production in Type ABs.

HIGHLY BENEFICIAL

Lentil (green)	Red bean
Miso*	Soy bean
Navy bean	Tempeh*
Pinto bean	Tofu*

*soy products

NEUTRAL

Cannellini bean	Snap bean
Copper bean	Soy cheese*
Green bean	Soy flakes*
Green pea	Soy granules*
Jícama bean	Soy milk*
Lentil (domestic, red)	String bean
Northern bean	Tamarind bean
Pea pod	White bean

*soy products

AVOID

Adzuki bean	Garbanzo bean (chickpea)
Black bean	Kidney bean
Black-eyed pea	Lima bean
Broad bean	Mung bean (sprouts)
Fava bean	

CHAPTER SEVEN

Grains, Breads and Pasta

BLOOD TYPE AB		Weekly, if your ancestry is . . .		
Grains, breads, and pasta	PORTION ½ cup dry grains/ pasta, 1 muffin, 2 slices bread	AFRICAN 6–8 x	CAUCASIAN 6–9 x	ASIAN 6–10 x

Generally, Type ABs do well on grains, but you need to limit your wheat consumption, especially if you have a pronounced mucous condition caused by asthma or frequent infections. Oatmeal, soy flakes, millet, farina, rice and soy granules are good Type AB choices, as are Essene and Ezekiel breads. Avoid buckwheat and corn.

You will benefit from a diet rich in rice rather than pasta, although you may have semolina or spinach pasta once or twice a week. Again, avoid corn and buckwheat in favor of oats and rye. Limit your intake of bran and wheat germ to once a week.

HIGHLY BENEFICIAL

Amaranth	Rice (white/brown/ basmati/wild)
Essene bread	Rice (puffed)
Ezekiel 4:9 bread (100 percent sprouted)	Rye bread (100 percent)
Millet	Ry-krisp
Oat bran	Rye flour
Oat flour	Rye vita
Oatmeal	Soy flour bread
Rice bran	Spelt (whole)
Rice bread	Wheat bread, sprouted (not essene/ezekiel)
Rice cake	

NEUTRAL

Barley	Cream of Wheat
Couscous (cracked wheat)	Familia
Cream of Rice	Farina

NEUTRAL (CONTINUED)

Gluten flour	Spinach pasta
Grape-Nuts	Wheat bran
Matzo	Wheat bran muffin
Quinoa	Wheat (gluten flour products)
Semolina pasta	Wheat (white flour products)
Seven grain bread/cereal	Wheat (whole wheat products)
Shredded wheat	Wheat germ
Spelt bread	

AVOID

Artichoke pasta (pure)	Cornmeal
Buckwheat/kasha	Grits
Corn (white/yellow/blue)	Kamut
Cornbread or muffin	Popcorn
Cornflakes	Soba noodles (100 percent buckwheat)

AVOID (CONTINUED)

Sorghum	Teff
Tapioca	Wheat (refined unbleached)

CHAPTER EIGHT

Vegetables

BLOOD TYPE AB		Daily, if your ancestry is . . .		
	PORTION	AFRICAN	CAUCASIAN	ASIAN
Cooked	1 cup, prepared	3–5 x	3–5 x	3–5 x
Raw	1 cup, prepared	3–5 x	3–5 x	3–5 x

Fresh vegetables are an important source of phyto-chemicals, the natural substances in foods that help prevent cancer and heart disease—diseases that afflict Type ABs more often as a result of weaker immune systems. You have a wide selection of vegetables that are good for you.

HIGHLY BENEFICIAL

Alfalfa sprouts	Broccoli
Beets	Cabbage juice
Beet greens	Carrot juice

HIGHLY BENEFICIAL (CONTINUED)

Cauliflower	Kale
Celery/juice	Mushroom, maitake
Collard greens	Mustard greens
Cucumber	Parsley
Dandelion	Parsnip
Eggplant	Potato, sweet
Garlic	Yam

NEUTRAL

Arugula	Chicory
Asparagus	Coriander leaf (cilantro)
Bamboo shoot	Cucumber juice
Bok choy	Daikon
Brussels sprouts	Endive
Cabbage, all kinds	Escarole
Carrot	Fennel
Celeriac	Fiddlehead fern

NEUTRAL (CONTINUED)

Ginger	Poi
Horseradish	Potato, red and white
Kohlrabi	Pumpkin
Leek	Rappini (broccoli rabe)
Lettuce, all kinds	Rutabaga
Mushroom, enoki	Sauerkraut
Mushroom, oyster	Scallion
Mushroom, portobello	Seaweed
Mushroom, silver dollar	Shallot
Mushroom, tree	Snow pea
Okra	Spinach/juice
Olive, Greek	Squash, all types
Olive, green	String bean
Olive, Spanish	Swiss chard
Onion, all types	Taro
Pea (green, pod)	Tomato/juice
Pimiento	Turnip

NEUTRAL (CONTINUED)

Water chestnut	Yucca
Watercress	Zucchini

AVOID

Aloe (tea, juice, leaves)	Olive, black
Artichoke, all types	Peppers, all types
Avocado	Pickles, all types
Corn	Radish (red)
Mushroom, abalone	Sprouts, mung
Mushroom, shiitake	Sprouts, radish

CHAPTER NINE

Fruits

BLOOD TYPE AB		Daily, if your ancestry is . . .		
Recommended fruits	PORTION 3–5 oz. or 1 fruit	AFRICAN 3–4 x	CAUCASIAN 3–4 x	ASIAN 3–4 x

Type ABs should emphasize the more alkaline fruits, such as grapes, plums, and berries. Avoid oranges, which are a stomach irritant for Type ABs, and also interfere with the absorption of important minerals. Lemons are also excellent for Type ABs, helping to aid digestion and clear mucus from the system. Since vitamin C is an important antioxidant, especially for stomach cancer prevention, eat other vitamin C–rich fruits, such as grapefruit or kiwi. The banana lectin interferes with Type AB digestion. I recommend substituting other high-potassium fruits such as apricots, figs, and certain melons.

HIGHLY BENEFICIAL

Cherry	Kiwi
Cranberry/juice	Lemon/juice
Fig, fresh/dried	Loganberry
Gooseberry	Pineapple
Grape, all types	Plum
Grapefruit	Watermelon

NEUTRAL

Apple cider/juice	Casaba melon
Apricot/juice	Christmas melon
Asian pear	Crenshaw melon
Blackberry/juice	Currants (black/red)
Blueberry	Date, all types
Boysenberry	Elderberry
Breadfruit	Grapefruit juice
Canang melon	Honeydew
Cantaloupe	Kumquat

NEUTRAL (CONTINUED)

Lime/juice	Plantain
Mulberry	Prune/juice
Mush melon	Raisin
Nectarine/juice	Raspberry
Papaya	Spanish melon
Peach	Strawberry
Pear/juice	Tangerine/juice
Pineapple juice	Youngberry

AVOID

Banana	Orange
Bitter melon	Persimmon
Coconut	Pomegranate
Dewberry	Prickly pear
Guava/juice	Quince
Loganberry	Sago palm
Mango/juice	Starfruit (carambola)

CHAPTER TEN

Juices and Fluids

BLOOD TYPE AB		Daily, if your ancestry is . . .		
	PORTION	AFRICAN	CAUCASIAN	ASIAN
Recommended juices	8 oz.	2–3 x	2–3 x	2–3 x
Water	8 oz.	4–7 x	4–7 x	4–7 x

Type ABs should begin each day by drinking a glass of warm water with the freshly squeezed juice of one-half lemon to cleanse your system of mucus that formed while you were sleeping. The lemon water also aids elimination. Follow with a diluted glass of grapefruit or papaya juice. Choose vegetables and fruits according to the recommendations in chapters 10 and 11 when making or buying juice. Stress highly alkaline fruit juices like black cherry, cranberry, or grape.

CHAPTER ELEVEN

Spices

Sea salt and kelp should be used in place of salt. Their
sodium content is low, and kelp has immensely positive
heart and immune system benefits. It is also useful for
weight control. Avoid all pepper and vinegar because
they are acidic. Instead of vinegar, use lemon juice with
oil and herbs to dress vegetables or salads. And don't be
afraid to use generous amounts of garlic. It's a potent
tonic and natural antibiotic, especially for Type ABs.
Sugar and chocolate are allowed in small amounts. Use
them as you would condiments.

HIGHLY BENEFICIAL

Curry	Miso
Garlic	Parsley
Horseradish	

NEUTRAL

Agar	Cream of tartar
Apple pectin	Cumin
Arrowroot	Dill
Basil	Dulse
Bay leaf	Honey
Bergamot	Juniper
Caper	Kelp
Caraway	Licorice root
Cardamom	Mace
Carob	Maple syrup
Chervil	Marjoram
Chili powder	Molasses
Chive	Mustard (dry)
Chocolate	Nutmeg
Cinnamon	Paprika
Clove	Peppermint
Coriander	Rice syrup

NEUTRAL (CONTINUED)

Rosemary	Tamari
Saffron	Tamarind
Sage	Tarragon
Savory	Thyme
Sea salt	Turmeric
Senna	Vanilla
Soy sauce	Wintergreen
Spearmint	Yeast (baker's/brewer's)
Sugar (white/brown)	

AVOID

Allspice	Cornstarch
Almond extract	Corn syrup
Anise	Dextrose
Aspartame	Fructose
Barley malt	Gelatin, plain
Carrageenan	Guarana

AVOID (CONTINUED)

Gums (Arabic, acacia)	Sucanat
Maltodextrin	Tapioca
Pepper, all types	Vinegar, all types

CHAPTER TWELVE

Condiments

Avoid all pickled condiments, due to a susceptibility to stomach cancer. Also avoid ketchup, which contains vinegar, and Worcestershire sauce, which contains corn syrup.

HIGHLY BENEFICIAL

None	

NEUTRAL

Jam (from acceptable fruits)	Mayonnaise
Jelly (from acceptable fruits)	Mustard

NEUTRAL (CONTINUED)

Salad dressing (from acceptable ingredients)	

AVOID

Ketchup	Pickles
Pickle relish	Worcestershire sauce

CHAPTER THIRTEEN

Herbs and Herbal Teas

Herbal tea should be employed by Type AB to rev up your immune system and build your protections against cardiovascular disease and cancer. Alfalfa, aloe, burdock, chamomile, and echinacea are immune system boosters. Hawthorn and licorice root are highly recommended for cardiovascular health. Green tea has enormous positive effect on the immune system. Dandelion, burdock root, and strawberry leaf teas will aid your absorption of iron and prevent anemia.

HIGHLY BENEFICIAL

Alfalfa	Echinacea
Burdock	Ginseng
Chamomile	Ginger

HIGHLY BENEFICIAL (CONTINUED)

Hawthorn	Rose hip
Licorice root	Strawberry leaf

NEUTRAL

Catnip	Sage
Cayenne	Sarsaparilla
Chickweed	Slippery elm
Dandelion	Spearmint
Dong quai	St. John's wort
Elder	Thyme
Goldenseal	Valerian
Horehound	Vervain
Mulberry	White birch
Parsley	White oak bark
Peppermint	Yarrow
Raspberry leaf	Yellow dock

AVOID

Aloe	Mullein
Coltsfoot	Red clover
Corn silk	Rhubarb
Fenugreek	Senna
Gentian	Shepherd's purse
Hops	Skullcap
Linden	

CHAPTER FOURTEEN

Miscellaneous Beverages

Red wine is good for Type ABs because of its positive cardiovascular effects. A glass of red wine every day is believed to lower the risk of heart disease for both men and women. Green tea has enormous positive effects on the immune system.

HIGHLY BENEFICIAL

Green tea	Red wine

NEUTRAL

Beer	White wine
Seltzer water	

AVOID

Coffee (regular/decaf)	Soda, all types
Liquor	Tea (black, regular, decaf)

CHAPTER FIFTEEN

Type AB Supplement Advisory

Your Type AB Plan also includes recommendations about vitamin, mineral, and herbal supplements that can enhance the effects of your diet. As with food, nutritional supplements don't always work the same way for everyone. Every vitamin, mineral, and herbal supplement plays a specific role in your body. The miracle remedy your Type O or Type B friend raves about may be inert or even harmful for your Type AB system.

Your goal for any kind of supplementation is to enhance your Type AB strengths and add an additional barrier of protection against your weaknesses. Therefore, your targeted focus should be:

- Supercharging your immune system.

- Supplying cancer-fighting antioxidants.

- Strengthening your heart.

The following recommendations emphasize the supplements that help to meet these goals, and also warn against the supplements that can be counterproductive or dangerous for Type ABs.

Type ABs get plenty of vitamin A, vitamin B_{12}, niacin, and vitamin E in in their diets, supplying a dietary protection against cancer and heart disease. I would suggest further supplementation only if, for some reason, a Type AB isn't adhering to the diet.

BENEFICIAL

Vitamin C

Type ABs, with naturally higher rates of stomach cancer, can benefit from taking additional supplements of vitamin C. As an antioxidant, vitamin C is known to protect against cancer. However, don't take this to mean that you should take massive amounts. I have found that Type ABs do not do as well on high doses (1000 mg and up) of vitamin C because it tends to upset their stomachs. Taken over the course of a day, two to four capsules of a 250 mg supplement, preferably derived from rose hips, should cause no digestive problems.

BEST C-RICH FOODS FOR TYPE ABS:
berries
broccoli
cherries
grapefruit
lemon
pineapple

Zinc [with caution]

I have found that a small amount of zinc supplementation (as little as 3 mg/day) often makes a big difference in protecting Type AB children against infections, especially ear infections. However, while small, periodic doses enhance immunity, long-term, higher doses depress it and can interfere with the absorption of other minerals. Be careful with zinc! It's completely unregulated and is widely available as a supplement, but you really shouldn't use it without a physician's advice.

BEST ZINC-RICH FOODS FOR TYPE ABS:

eggs
_____

legumes
_____

recommended meats
(especially dark meat turkey)
_____

HERBS/PHYTOCHEMICALS

Hawthorn (*Crataegus oxyacantha*). With a tendency toward heart disease, Type ABs can benefit from hawthorn, a phytochemical with exceptional preventive capacities. Hawthorn increases the elasticity of the arteries and strengthens the heart while also lowering blood pressure and exerting a mild solventlike effect upon the plaque in the arteries.

Immune-enhancing herbs. Because the immune system of Type AB tends to be vulnerable to viruses and infections, gentle immune-enhancing herbs such as purple coneflower (*Echinacea purpurea*) can help to ward off colds or flus and may help optimize the immune system's anticancer surveillance.

Calming herbs. Type ABs can benefit from mild herbal relaxants such as chamomile and valerian root. These herbs are available as teas and should be taken frequently.

Quercetin. Quercetin is a very powerful antioxidant, many hundreds of times more powerful than vitamin E. Quercetin makes a powerful addition to your cancer-prevention strategies.

Milk thistle (*Silybum marianum*). Milk thistle is an effective antioxidant with the additional special property of reaching very high concentrations in the liver and bile ducts. Type ABs tend to suffer from digestive disorders, particularly of the liver and gallbladder. If your family has any history of liver, pancreas, or gallbladder problems, add a milk thistle supplement. Cancer patients receiving chemotherapy should use a milk thistle supplement to protect their livers from damage.

Bromelain (pineapple enzymes). If you suffer from bloating or other signs of poor absorption, take a bromelain supplement. This enzyme has a moderate ability to break down dietary proteins, helping the Type AB digestive tract better assimilate proteins.

CHAPTER SIXTEEN

Medical Strategies

Modern science has presented the medical community with a bewildering array of medications, and all of them are being prescribed by well-meaning physicians world-wide. But have we been careful enough in our use of an-tibiotics and vaccines? How do you know which medications are best for you, for your family, for your children? Again, blood type holds the answer.

As a naturopathic physician, I try to avoid prescribing over-the-counter medications. In most cases, there are natural alternatives that work just as well or better—and they don't have some of the problematic side effects of many pharmaceutical preparations.

The following natural remedies are safe for Type AB:

ARTHRITIS

alfalfa

boswellia

calcium

Epsom salt bath

rosemary tea soak

CONGESTION

licorice tea

mullein

nettle

vervain

CONSTIPATION

fiber

larch tree bark (ARA-6)

psyllium

slippery elm

COUGH

coltsfoot

horehound

linden

CRAMPS, GAS

chamomile tea

fennel tea

ginger

peppermint tea

probiotic supplement with bifidus factor

DIARRHEA

blueberries

elderberries

L. acidophilus (yogurt culture)

raspberry leaf

EARACHE

garlic-mullein-olive-oil eardrops

FEVER

feverfew

vervain

white willow bark

catnip

FLU

echinacea

elderberry (prevention)

garlic

goldenseal

arabinogalactan

rose hip tea

HEADACHE

chamomile

feverfew

valerian

white willow bark

INDIGESTION, HEARTBURN

bromelain

ginger

goldenseal

peppermint

MENSTRUAL CRAMPS

Jamaican dogwood

NAUSEA

ginger

licorice root tea

cayenne

SINUSITIS

thyme

SORE THROAT

goldenseal-root-and-sage-tea gargle

TOOTHACHE

crushed-garlic gum massage

oil-of-cloves gum massage

CHAPTER SEVENTEEN

Frequently Asked Questions

Do I have to make all of the changes at once for my Type AB Diet to work?

No. On the contrary, I suggest you start slowly, gradually eliminating the foods that are not good for you and increasing those that are highly beneficial. Many diet programs urge you to plunge in headfirst and radically change your life immediately. I think it's more realistic and ultimately more effective if you engage in a learning process. Don't just take my word for it. You have to "learn" it in your body. Before you begin your Type AB Diet, you may know very little about which foods are good or bad for you. You're used to making your choices according to your taste buds, family traditions, and fad diet books. Chances are you are eating some foods that are good for you, but the Type AB Diet provides you with a powerful tool for making informed choices every time. Once you know what your optimal eating plan is, you have the freedom to veer from your diet on occasion. Rigidity is the enemy of joy; I certainly am not a proponent of it. The Type AB Diet is designed to make you feel great, not miserable and deprived. Obviously, there are going to be times when common sense tells you to relax the rules a bit—such as when you're eating at a relative's house.

I'm Blood Type AB and my husband is Blood Type O. How do we cook and eat together? I don't want to prepare two separate meals.

My wife, Martha, and I have exactly the same situation. Martha is Type O and I am Type A. We find that we can usually share about two-thirds of a meal. The main difference is in the protein source. For example, if we make a stir-fry, Martha might separately prepare some chicken while I'll add cooked tofu. Or if we're eating a pasta dish, Martha might add a little cooked ground beef to her portion. It has become relatively easy for us because we are quite familiar with the specifics of each other's Blood Type Diet. I suggest you refer to the comprehensive books *Eat Right 4 Your Type* and *Cook Right 4 Your Type* for information and suggestions for living happily in multiple blood type families. I know that people often worry that there might be too many differences between blood types to make it work. But think about it. There are over 200 foods listed for each diet—many of them compatible across the board. Considering that the average person only eats about 25 foods, the Blood Type Diets actually offer more, not fewer, options.

Why do you list different portion recommendations according to ancestry?

The portions listings according to ancestry are merely refinements to the diet that you may find helpful. In the same way that men, women, and children have different portion standards, so, too, do people according to their body size and weight, geography, and cultural food preferences. These suggestions will help you get started until you are comfortable enough with the diet to naturally eat the appropriate portions. The portion recommendations also take into account specific problems that people of different ancestries tend to have with food. African-Americans, for example, are often lactose intolerant, and most Asians are unaccustomed to eating dairy foods, so they may have to introduce these foods slowly to avoid negative reactions.

Must I eat all of the foods marked "highly beneficial"?

It would be impossible to eat everything on your diet! Think of your Blood Type Diet as a painter's palette from which you may choose colors in different shades and combinations. However, do try to reach the weekly amount of the various food groups, if possible. Frequency is probably more important than the individual portions. If you have a small build, reduce the size of your portions, but maintain a regular frequency. This will ensure that the most valuable nutrients will continue to be delivered into the blood stream at a constant rate.

What should I do if an "avoid" food is the fourth or fifth ingredient in a recipe?

That depends on the severity of your condition, or the degree of your compliance. If you have food allergies, or colitis, you may want to practice complete avoidance. Many high-compliance patients avoid these foods altogether, although I think this might be too extreme. Unless you suffer from a specific allergic condition, it won't hurt most people to occasionally eat a food that is not on their diet.

Will I lose weight on the Blood Type Diet?

There are several ways to answer that question. First, most people who are overweight are eating an imbalanced diet—foods that upset metabolism, hamper proper digestion, and cause water retention. These are all factors that lead to overweight. The Blood Type Diet is the ultimate *balanced* diet, specifically tailored for you. If you follow your Blood Type Diet, your metabolism will adjust to its normal level and you'll burn calories more efficiently; your digestive system will process nutrients properly and reduce water retention. In time, perhaps a very short time, your weight will adjust accordingly. In my practice, I've found that most of my patients who have weight problems also have a history of chronic dieting. One would think that constant dieting would lead to weight loss, but that's not true if the structure of the diet and the foods it includes go against everything that makes sense for your specific body type. In our culture, we tend to promote "one size fits all" weight-loss programs, and then we wonder why they don't work. The answer is obvious! Different blood types respond to food in different ways.

Do calories matter on the Blood Type Diet?

There is an adjustment period on this diet, and over time you'll be able to adjust food amounts according to your needs. It's important to be aware of portion sizes. No matter *what* you eat, if you eat *too much* of it you'll gain weight. This probably seems so obvious that it doesn't even bear mentioning. But overeating has become one of America's most difficult and dangerous health problems. Millions of Americans are bloated and dyspeptic because of the amounts of food they eat. When you eat excessively, the walls of your stomach stretch like an inflated balloon. Although stomach muscles are elastic and were created to contract and expand, when they are grossly enlarged the cells of the abdominal walls undergo a tremendous strain. If you are eating until you feel full, and you normally feel sluggish after a meal, try to reduce your portion sizes. Learn to listen to what your body is telling you.

I've never heard of many of the grains you mention. Where do I find out more?

If you're looking for alternative grains, health food stores are a bonanza. In recent years, many ancient grains, largely forgotten, have been rediscovered and are now being produced. Examples of these are amaranth, a grain from Mexico, and spelt, a variation of wheat that seems to be free of the problems found with whole wheat. Try them! They're not bad. Spelt flour makes a hearty, chewy bread that is quite flavorful, while several interesting breakfast cereals are now being made with amaranth. Another alternative is to use sprouted wheat breads, some-times referred to as "Ezekiel" or "Essene" bread, as the gluten lectins found principally in the seed coat are de-stroyed by the sprouting process. These breads spoil rap-idly and are usually found in the refrigerator cases of health-food stores. They are a "live" food, with many ben-eficial enzymes still intact. (Beware of commercially pro-duced "sprouted wheat" breads, as they usually have a minority of sprouted wheat and a majority of whole wheat in their formulas.) Sprouted wheat breads are somewhat sweet tasting, as the sprouting process also releases sug-ars, and are moist and chewy. They make wonderful toast.

I'm allergic to peanuts, but you say they're a highly beneficial food for Type AB.

Let me suggest that you reevaluate whether you really do have an allergy to peanuts, since allergic reactions are usually caused by lectins that react badly to your blood type. It may be that you think you're allergic to peanuts because you had a negative experience with them once, or someone told you that you had an allergy. Doctors and laypeople alike tend to assume there are allergies when they don't have good explanations for problems. It may be that for you peanuts were just a convenient scapegoat for reactions you were having to other foods.

Type AB at a Glance

TYPE AB
The Enigma
rare · versatile · spiritual

STRENGTHS	WEAKNESSES	MEDICAL RISKS
Designed for modern conditions	Sensitive digestive tract	Heart disease
		Cancer
	Open to microbial invasion	
Highly tolerant immune system		
Versatile		

DIET PROFILE	WEIGHT LOSS KEY	SUPPLEMENTS	EXERCISE REGIMEN
MIXED DIET	AVOID	Vitamin C	Calming,
	Chicken	Hawthorn	centering
Meat	Corn	Echinacea	exercises,
Fish	Kidney	Valerian	such as
Dairy	beans	Quercetin	yoga,
Tofu	Buckwheat	Milk thistle	combined
Beans			with
Legumes	USE		moderate
Grains	Tofu		exercise,
Vegetables	Seafood		such as
Fruits	Greens		cycling and
	Kelp		tennis

Blood Type Learning Center

Now that you're familiar with the basic principles of the Blood Type Diet, I encourage you to expand your level of learning and application. The "right for your type" series offers the most comprehensive, scientifically grounded, and clinically tested information available on the four blood types. In order to truly make the most of your individualized diet and lifestyle recommendations, it's important for you to have a working knowledge of all four blood types. Your differences do not exist in a vacuum, but are part of nature's complex system of opposition and synergism. Your understanding of the evolutionary factors that distinguish the blood types will enhance your ability to live more fully as a Type AB. In addition, these books offer extensive additional information and recommendations about your blood type. The series includes:

Live Right 4 Your Type
The Individualized Prescription for
Maximizing Health, Metabolism, and
Vitality in Every Stage of Your Life
by Dr. Peter J. D'Adamo, with Catherine Whitney
(G. P. Putnam's Sons, 2001)
Also available on audiocassette

In *Live Right 4 Your Type*, Dr. D'Adamo shows how living according to blood type can help people achieve total physical and emotional health at every stage of life. Aided by cutting-edge genetic research and the documentation of hundreds of research studies, Dr. D'Adamo presents readers with a life-enhancing program, which includes:

- The latest discoveries about the genetics of blood type and how they affect the body's systems.

- A study of the role of subtypes, in particular secretor status.

- Groundbreaking data on the connection between blood type and stress, personality, and mental health.

- A thorough investigation of the variations in digestion, metabolism, and immunity, depending on blood type.

- Individualized blood type prescriptions that show how to make lifestyle adaptations, reduce stress, gain emotional balance, slow down aging, and avoid disease.

- Targeted advice for children, seniors, and women.

- Extensive research notes, patient outcomes, and resources.

Eat Right 4 Your Type
The Individualized Diet Solution to
Staying Healthy, Living Longer &
Achieving Your Ideal Weight
by Dr. Peter J. D'Adamo, with Catherine Whitney
(G. P. Putnam's Sons, 1996)
Also available on audiocassette

Eat Right 4 Your Type is Dr. D'Adamo's ground-breaking book, which first introduced the concept of the connection between blood type, diet and health to a mass audience. With over two million copies in print and translated into fifty languages, *Eat Right 4 Your Type* remains the seminal work in the field. It includes:

- A detailed exploration of the anthropological and biological origins of the blood types.

- Comprehensive diet, exercise and meal plans for each blood type.

- Special recommendations for medical problems, weight loss, aging, infertility, and other issues.

- Case histories from Dr. D'Adamo's clinic, showing the remarkable results of the Blood Type Diet.

- An extensive bibliography, research and support section.

Cook Right 4 Your Type
The Practical Kitchen Companion to
Eat Right 4 Your Type
by Dr. Peter J. D'Adamo, with Catherine Whitney
(G. P. Putnam's Sons, 1998)

Cook Right 4 Your Type is the essential guide for living with and enjoying your Blood Type Diet. With the assistance of a team of professional chefs, Dr. D'Adamo presents a book chock full of vital information and delicious recipes for each blood type. The book features:

- Food lists and shopping guides to help you set up your kitchen.

- Family-friendly recipe charts that show how to cook for more than one blood type.

- Hundreds of tips and practical guidelines for eating right for your type.

- 30-day meal plans to help integrate the diet into daily life.

- More than 200 original recipes to please every blood type palate.

Resources and Support

DR. PETER J. D'ADAMO: PATIENT SERVICES

Dr. Peter D'Adamo and his staff continue to accept new patients on a limited basis. To find out more about scheduling an appointment, please contact:

Dr. Peter D'Adamo, ND, MIfHI
Chief Medical Officer
Center for Personalized Medicine
213 Danbury Road
Wilton, CT 06897
Phone: 203 834 7500
Fax: 203 834 7504
http://www.dadamo.com/clinic/

Note: Please do not submit questions regarding Dr. D'Adamo's work or seeking personal advice on health matters.

ON THE WEB: WWW.DADAMO.COM

The World Wide Web has proven to be a valuable venue for exploring and applying the tenets of the Blood Type Diet and lifestyle. Since January 1997 hundreds of thousands have visited the site to participate in the ABO chat groups, to peruse the scientific archives, to share experiences and recipes, and to learn more about the science of blood type. The Web site has an interactive message board and archives of past posts to the board.

One of the most important features on the Web page is the Results Database, which has facilitated the collection of data on the measurable effects of the Blood Type Diet on a wide range of medical conditions. Visitors are encouraged to share their results.

SELF-TESTING SERVICES

North American Pharmacal, Inc, is the official distributor of Home Blood Type Testing Kits. Each kit costs $9.95 and is a single-use disposable educational device capable of determining one individual's ABO and rhesus blood type. Results are obtained within about four to five minutes. If you have several friends or family members who need to learn their blood type, you will need to order a separate home blood-typing kit for each individual.

If you are ordering a kit to be shipped outside of the U.S., shipping rates can vary dramatically and can be quite expensive. Please contact our customer service department prior to placing your order for an estimate of shipping charges for non-U.S. orders, or visit the Web site in your region.

D'Adamo Personalized Nutrition
North American Pharmacal, Inc.
213 Danbury Road
Wilton, CT 06897
Phone: 203 761 0042
Fax: 203 761 0043
www.4yourtype.com

North American Pharmacal, Inc., offers a range of other self-tests to monitor aspects of health such as stress hormone levels, female hormone levels, mineral balance, and antioxidant status. There is also a test to determine secretor status. For prices and ordering information please contact North American Pharmacal or visit the Web site.

BLOOD TYPE PRODUCTS AND SUPPLEMENTS

North American Pharmacal, Inc., is the official distributor of Blood Type Specialty Products. The product line includes supplements, books, videos, teas, meal replacement bars, cosmetics, and support material that makes eating and living right for your type easier. Included in this product line are: New Chapter® D'Adamo 4 Your Type Products™. These whole-food vitamins, herbs, and other food supplements have been specifically crafted to address the unique requirements of each blood type.

Also included are Sip Right 4 Your Type™ teas, Deflect™ lectin-blocking formulas, and a range of additional blood-type-specific and blood-type-friendly health products that have been formulated in partnership with The Republic of Tea and New Chapter.

Dr. Peter D'Adamo's official distributors in the UK can be contacted at:

NAP4EU Ltd
59 Bridge Street
Dollar
Clackmannanshire
FK14 7DQ
Scotland

Tel: +44 1259 743200
Email: info@right4eu.com
www.right4eu.com

He just wanted a decent book to read ...

Not too much to ask, is it? It was in 1935 when Allen Lane, Managing Director of Bodley Head Publishers, stood on a platform at Exeter railway station looking for something good to read on his journey back to London. His choice was limited to popular magazines and poor-quality paperbacks – the same choice faced every day by the vast majority of readers, few of whom could afford hardbacks. Lane's disappointment and subsequent anger at the range of books generally available led him to found a company – and change the world.

'We believed in the existence in this country of a vast reading public for intelligent books at a low price, and staked everything on it'
Sir Allen Lane, 1902–1970, founder of Penguin Books

The quality paperback had arrived – and not just in bookshops. Lane was adamant that his Penguins should appear in chain stores and tobacconists, and should cost no more than a packet of cigarettes.

Reading habits (and cigarette prices) have changed since 1935, but Penguin still believes in publishing the best books for everybody to enjoy. We still believe that good design costs no more than bad design, and we still believe that quality books published passionately and responsibly make the world a better place.

So wherever you see the little bird – whether it's on a piece of prize-winning literary fiction or a celebrity autobiography, political tour de force or historical masterpiece, a serial-killer thriller, reference book, world classic or a piece of pure escapism – you can bet that it represents the very best that the genre has to offer.

Whatever you like to read – trust Penguin.

read more
www.penguin.co.uk